Gym: A Beginner's Guide

Create the perfect programme for you.

Contents:

Failing to prepare is preparing to fail

Introduction

Is it better to work hard or work smart? Beginners tend to vastly underestimate the impact of proper planning on training. There is much more to getting in shape than randomly lifting weights. Whist this approach may work, it's far from optimal – it's best to have a plan. The aim of this book is to simplify the overwhelming amount of knowledge within the fitness industry and media to provide the novice gym-goer with simple, practical and effective advice for making gains.

In this generation, it's easier than ever for beginner lifters to innocently believe false claims made from the clouded fitness industry. Buying into these "bro-science" myths can be hugely detrimental to beginners and unfortunately, it's often difficult to know what to believe. There are still contentions over some aspects of training in the professional community, but this book is based on established scientific principles of programming and training.

As with all disciplines, mastery takes time. It is not necessary to spend hours in the gym every day, but it is important to understand that a physique is not built overnight, over a week, or even a month, but over years. The good news is that most of your genetic potential can be achieved within the first 2/3 years of training if done correctly, and these gains are much easier to maintain once they're made. Returns are diminishing when training for size and strength, which is why it's even more important to profit from the "beginner gains" period and establish good habits if training becomes more serious later in life.

Finding a random programme online or following a celebrity's programme is likely vastly different from what you require. This book aims to equip you with the relevant knowledge you need to design and follow an appropriate programme for you.

PART 1: Physical Wellbeing

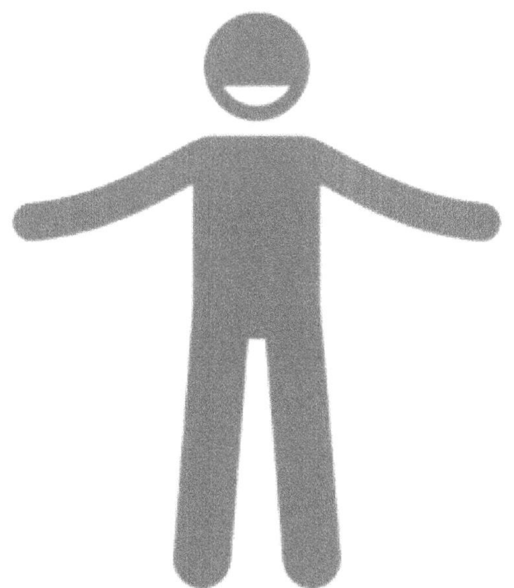

Components to a physical wellbeing

Lifting weights doesn't have to dictate your life. There are many aspects to a happy, healthy life and exercise is only part of that. The three pillars of physical wellbeing, in order of importance are:

Sleep

Nourishment

Physical activity

Mental wellbeing

It would be impossible to numerically rationalise how important each of these pillars are in relation to each other, however they are listed in order of priority. This book is about training which of course falls under activity however these components are mentioned to show that it is necessary to have the other two in place, in concordance with the last. You cannot expect to make great progress in the gym without paying attention to these supporting aspects - the better sleep and nutrition are, the better training will be. These pillars are all huge topics themselves, but here is a brief summary of the importance of each of them.

Mental wellbeing

Mental and physical wellbeing influence each other very much. A healthy body promotes a happy mind and vice versa. The physiologies behind mental wellbeing are too big to summaries here, but mental wellbeing will affect, and be affected by, the three pillars of physical health, which is why it encompasses them all above. To promote physical wellbeing, it is a good to minimise stress as much as possible. This will encourage the neurological and physical adaptations that promote muscle growth to occur, as well as boosting general mood. It is a good idea to schedule down time into daily life to combat stress.

Sleep

Sleep is when recovery (building muscle and gaining strength) takes place, so it is in the best interest of any athlete to optimise it. Good sleep offers a myriad of benefits and the importance of proper sleep hygiene is becoming increasingly widespread. Here are some guidelines, in order of importance, to promote good sleep:

1) Quantity – Allow ample opportunity for sleep every night. Eight hours is recommended, although this will differ between individuals.

2) Be consistent with sleep timings regardless of the day (weekday/weekend). The human body has evolved to rely on a circadian rhythm, so sleeping and waking regularly will ensure hormones are released at the correct time. There is no recommended time to sleep and wake – this will again depend on individual differences like age and chronotype.

3) Keep your bedroom dark and cool when sleeping and use it exclusively for sleep and sex.

4) Allow time to wind down by reducing activities that stimulate the mind, like gaming, before sleeping.

5) Avoid alcohol and caffeine in the afternoon. These substances stay in the body for a long time and whilst some may use alcohol to encourage sleep, like caffeine, it prevents natural sleep cycles.

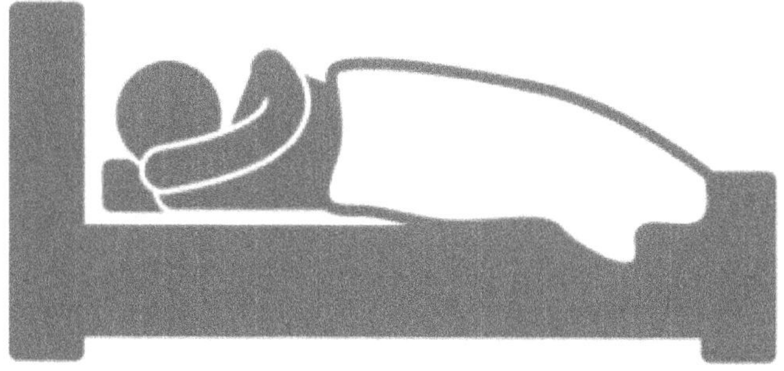

Nourishment and nutrition

There is also an overwhelming amount of information regarding nutrition out there, and with buzz words like "superfood" and "antioxidant" constantly headlining articles, it can be just as confusing as training itself. Here is a hierarchy pyramid of nutrition principles, where the bottom concept provides a foundation for the others, which decrease in importance up the pyramid:

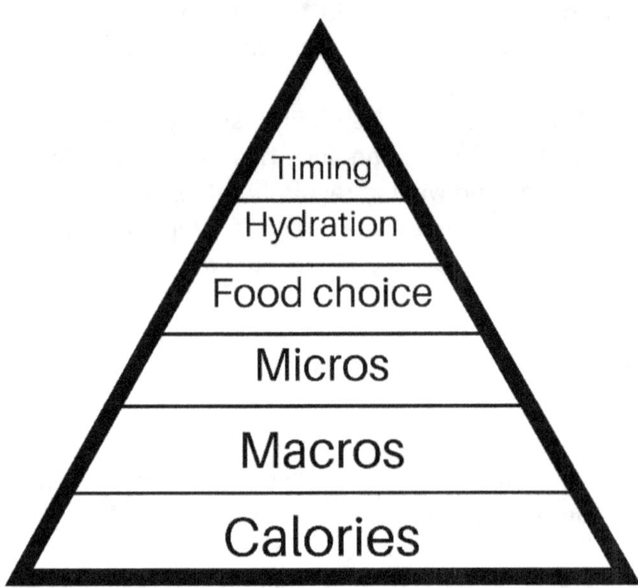

1) Calories – To gain weight, you must eat in a calorie surplus - that is eating more than you burn. To lose weight, you must eat in a calorie deficit - that is eating less than you burn. When attempting either of these feats, it is recommended to take an average weight over the course of a week and reweigh another average a few weeks later to see if the surplus or deficit is enough. In either case, a slow and gradual increase or decrease in calorie intake is better than making drastic changes. Start by adding or removing 150-300 calories and increase this surplus or deficit each week until you reach your goal.

It is easier to drink calories than it is to eat them. This can be used to a personal advantage when looking to gain or lose weight.

The question of whether to bulk and cut or make lean gains depends on the individual and their goals. Exact insights to these methods are not discussed here.

2) Macros: The three divisions of macronutrients are proteins, carbohydrates and fats. When gaining muscle, it is recommended to consume about 1g of protein per 1lb of body mass per day and spread the intake out over the course of the day to maximise protein synthesis. Macro split ratios will be different depending on individual goals.

3) Micros: Micronutrients are vitamins and minerals that are essential for bodily functions and are extremely important for recovery. Plentiful fruit, and more importantly vegetables, should be consumed – between 5-8 a day is a good target.

4) Food choice: There are new diet plans released all the time. A clean diet of mostly unprocessed, whole foods is more important than individual food choice. For the beginner athlete, a diet does not need to be 100% strict. An 80:20 split of clean, healthy foods to dirty, processed foods is a good target – bare this in mind if you plan on having "cheat days".

Microbiome in the gut is an increasingly popular topic of scientific research. Eating foods that promote the diversity of microbes in the gut is very healthy. A Mediterranean diet is a good example of such a diet.

5) Hydration: Stay hydrated by drinking plenty of water every day. This is important but is ranked low in the pyramid as it is very easy to do.

6) Chrononutrition/meal timing: A pre-workout meal/snack can help fuel a workout and a post workout meal rich in protein will help with recovery and muscle growth. Be aware of consuming caffeinated pre-workout products if you train in the late afternoon/evening as this will negatively affect sleep, which is much more important. Meal timing itself is not of great concern to a beginner, although it is recommended to eat meals at roughly the same time each day

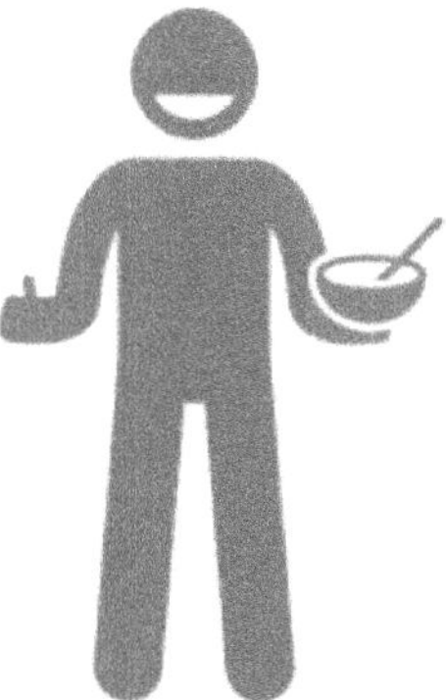

Simple tips for improving your diet

1) Make it sustainable and enjoyable: The best way to do this is to build up to a new diet plan rather than changing overnight. The best diet is one you can stick to, which will always be one you enjoy. There are plenty of enjoyable ways to eat healthily so just find what works for you rather than copying someone else's.

2) Use meal frequency to your advantage: For people trying to gain weight, eat more meals regularly throughout the day. For those looking to lose weight, intermittent fasting may be a better option.

3) Ignore supplementation: Most beginners think that having a scoop of a well-branded supplement each day is the answer to their dream physique. The truth is that even for more advanced athletes, most supplements are completely unnecessary. Don't buy into advertising and promotions; the only supplement a beginner should consider is quality whey protein to help hit daily protein targets. Most of your protein should however come from your food and with a good enough diet, even whey protein isn't necessary. A pre-workout supplement may be useful, but again is by no means essential.

4) Stay away from alcohol: Excessive alcohol (often considered the fourth macronutrient) is bad for the body. Not only does it negatively impact sleep, it is dehydrating and carries "dead calories" which provide no use to the body.

5) Don't overthink every detail: Eating well is unnecessarily overcomplicated. Unless you are committed to becoming a top-level athlete, you don't need to be too strict; just follow these guidelines.

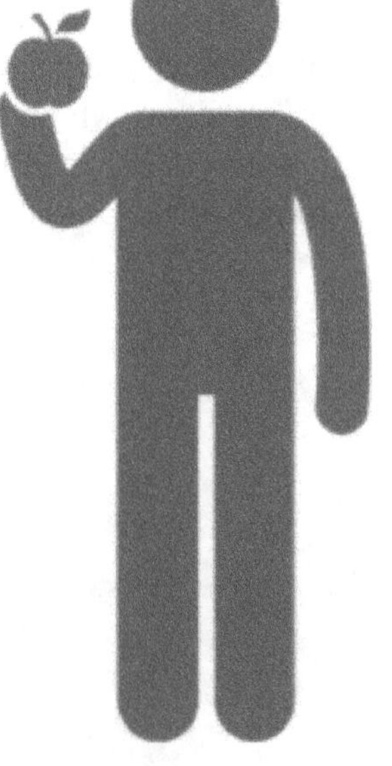

Physical activity

Lifting weights is a great way to maintain a physical active lifestyle. A completely sedentary lifestyle outside of gym however is still unhealthy. Vigorous hours of daily cardio are not necessary, however sitting down for hours at a time is unnatural and should be avoided as much as possible. If your job or lifestyle involves this kind of inactivity, taking regular breaks to move is a good idea.

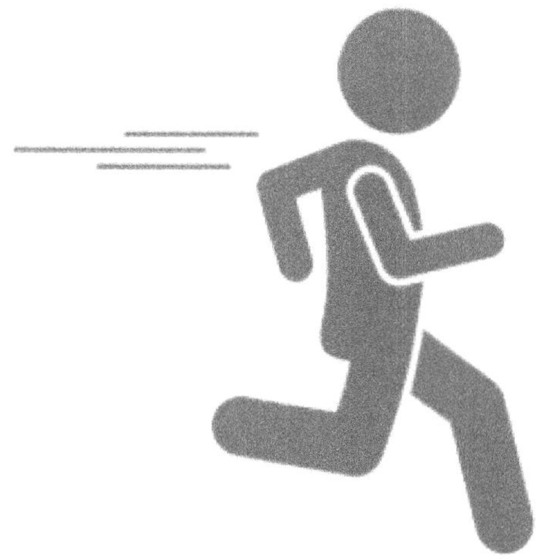

PART 2: Principles of Training

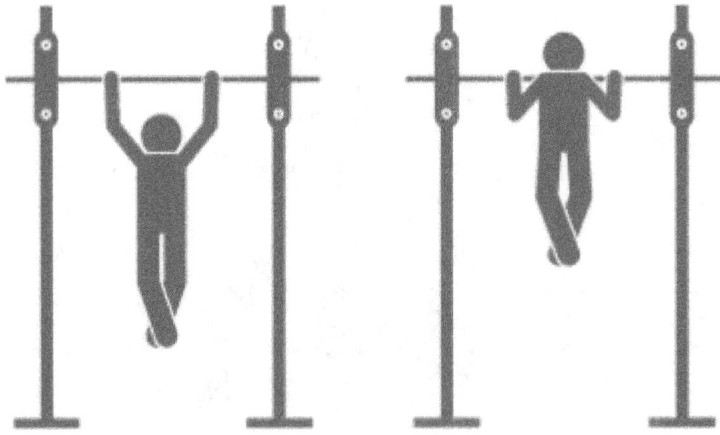

Overview

Making progress in the gym requires a solid programme and good programme execution. Programme design is covered in part 4 and execution in part 5.

There are many factors which determine the quality of a training programme but before considering the training variables, the general principles of training must be considered. Here is a hierarchy pyramid of training principles to consider.

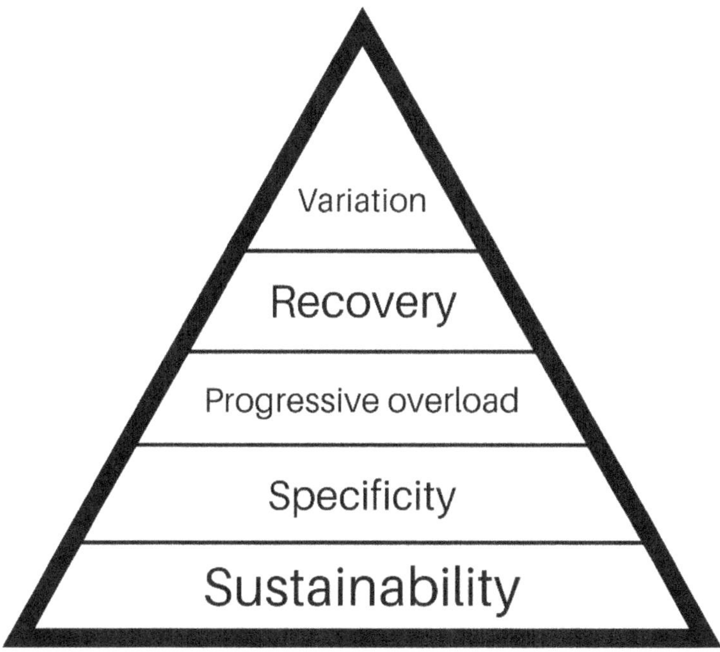

Sustainability:

As transformations like hypertrophy take time, any programme must be sustainable.

Application:

Training is made sustainable by 2 main factors:

-being safe – this is done by using proper form on exercises, which prevent injuries that would sabotage the process.

-being enjoyable - this is done by keeping it personal and setting realistic goals.

Specificity

There is no point designing the perfect programme if it isn't specific to your goals and personal lifestyle. Many people go to the gym to "get fit" however this is a very broad goal as there are many different components of fitness: strength, hypertrophy, endurance, flexibility, agility, skill and others. Whilst all these attributes could be trained simultaneously, little progress would be made in each, so it is much better to focus on one or two, at least periodically. Marathon runners and sprinters are both fit but train very differently as they require different skillsets. This book focusses on hypertrophy training, which overlaps with strength training.

It is important to set a realistic goal. This means accounting for individual differences like gender, age, and genetics. Lies told by social media influencers often promote unrealistic or even impossible goals so keep it personal and realistic. Creating easier, short-term goals as well as long term goals is a good idea.

Application:

Choose a specific goal. All the training variables (part 3) should be tailored to this goal

"Muscle toning" is a common goal for gym-goers. The only way tone muscles is by leaning out a physique, so to tone muscle, the goal should be fat loss - of course, bigger muscles will show more tone too.

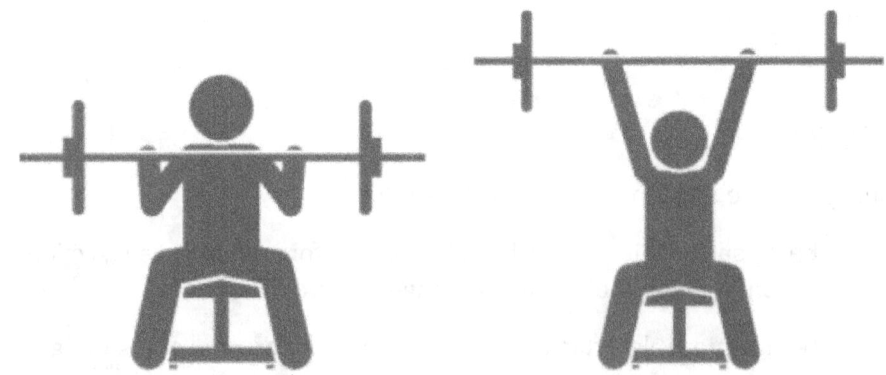

Progressive overload

An overloading stimulus will cause the body to adapt and improve. However, overtime the body becomes resistant to the stimulus and so it must become progressively more difficult in some way, imposing a greater stimulus each time. Training must always induce an overloading stimulus as the body becomes more resistant to it. This is done by manipulating the training variables, which are discussed in part 3.

<u>Application:</u>

Lifting weights provides an overloading stimulus. The supercompensation of adaptations that occur during recovery can promote strength, hypertrophic muscular endurance responses.

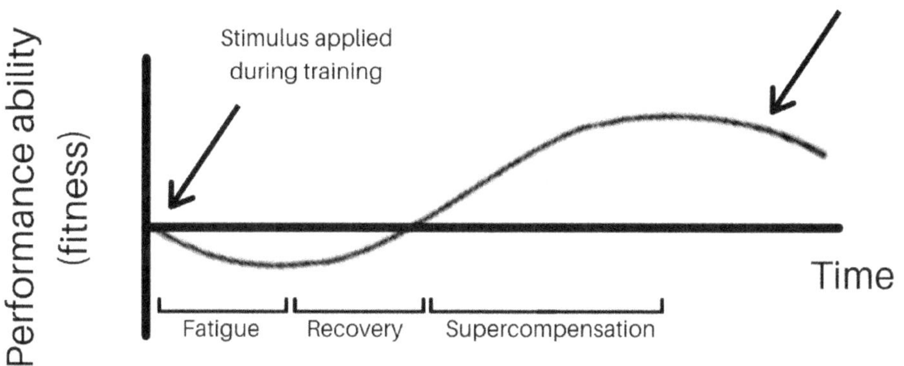

Undertraining occurs when performance level drops back to baseline before the next stimulus is applied, resulting in stagnation of performance ability.

Overtraining occurs when a second stimulus is applied before full recovery, resulting in a decline of performance ability.

It is generally agreed upon that the three hypertrophic mechanisms are mechanical tension, metabolic stress and muscle damage. Exact explanations of these mechanisms are outside the scope of this book.

Recovery:

As seen in the prior graph, fatigue is induced on the body as a stimulus is applied and so times of rest are needed to recover. Greater stimulus will result in greater supercompensation, however as it also means more fatigue, it is extremely important to balance recovery with the training stimulus. It is impossible to train with maximum stimulus frequently without a decline in performance (overtraining). Oppositely, it is important not to train too infrequently which will lead to undertraing. Fatigue must be regulated in concordance with stimulus.

<u>Application</u>

When training for strength and size, fatigue can be induced in many forms:

Local muscular fatigue - fatigue within the muscle group
being trained

Neurological fatigue – fatigue within the nervous system

Phycological fatigue – fatigue within the mind

Cardiovascular fatigue – fatigue within the cardiovascular system

Systemic fatigue – fatigue within the body as a whole (combination of
above)

All these types of fatigue relate to each other. It is important to understand that it is not possible to train with maximum intensity all the time. Periods of rest between sets, workouts and training blocks are required to accommodate this recovery, allowing fatigue to dissipate. Your programme should reflect these relevant recovery times.

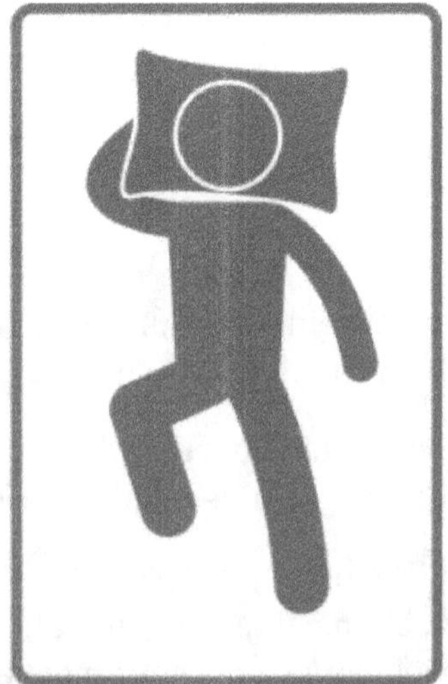

Variation:

To ensure an overload is progressive, some aspects of training must vary. Novelty in training is also a powerful way to combat the body's nature to become resistant to a stimulus we present it. The manipulation of the training variables is what makes or breaks a programme.

<u>Application</u>:

Variation is achieved by manipulating the training variables within a programme. This is discussed in the next section.

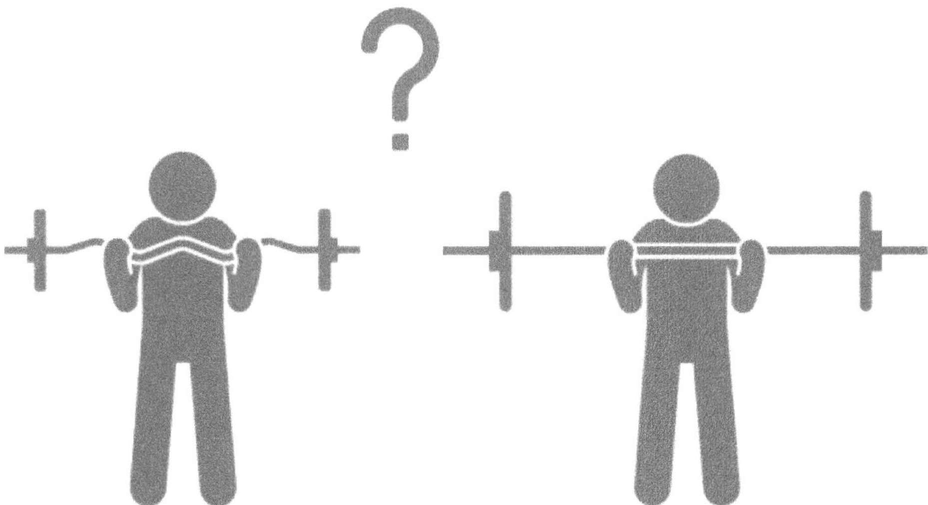

PART 3: Programme Considerations

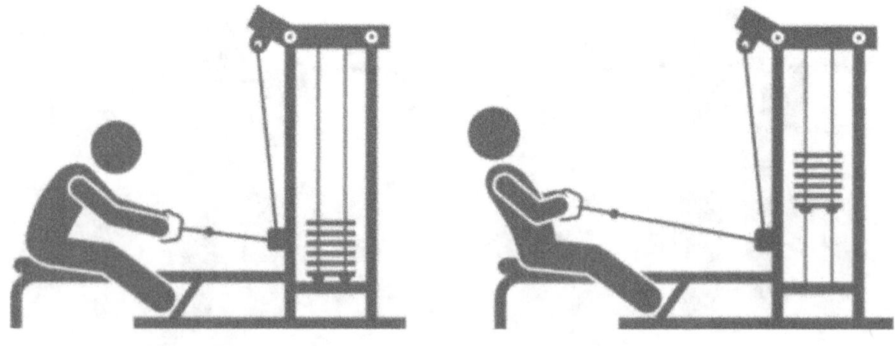

Definitions:

Rep (repetition): The number of repetitions of an exercise performed in a single set.

Set: Multiple repetitions performed consecutively between periods of rest.

Failure: The point at which no more reps can be performed with good form in a set (technical failure).

Intensity/load: The amount of weight being lifted during a set of an exercise. This can be expressed as a weight, or as a percentage of an individual's 1 rep max – the maximum load capable of being lifted for 1 repetition for a given exercise.

Volume: Total amount of work performed in a given time, usually a week. Sets x reps x load

Work capacity: The amount of volume an individual can regularly train and recover from.

There are over 600 muscles in the human body and no movement exclusively trains a single muscle, which is why the term muscle group is used instead of muscle; eg. chest rather that individuals chest muscles: pectoralis major, pectoralis minor etc. Muscle groups are sometimes subdivided; eg. upper chest, mid chest, lower chest.

Exercises can be split into two categories:

Compound exercises: Multi joint exercises that train multiple muscle groups simultaneously.

Isolation exercises: Single joint exercises that train single muscle groups.

Variation and periodisation:

Variation is implemented for two reasons: 1. It keeps the training stimulus fresh, preventing resilience of the body to adapt. 2. As overload must be progressive, variation of the training variables ensures the stimulus is constantly overloading. Therefore, it is important to balance the training variables properly, which is the challenge of programme design.

A training programme can be viewed in 3 different levels of scope, revealing 3 different cycles or "blocks" of training. Periodisation refers to the periodic manipulation of the training variables at any of these scope levels.

Microcycle: The shortest repeating block, typically one week long.

Mesocycle: A block of microcycles, typically 4/5 weeks long. A collection of mesocycles form a standard training programme.

Macrocycle: A block of mesocycles, lasting anywhere from 6-12 months. This usually contains different training programmes.

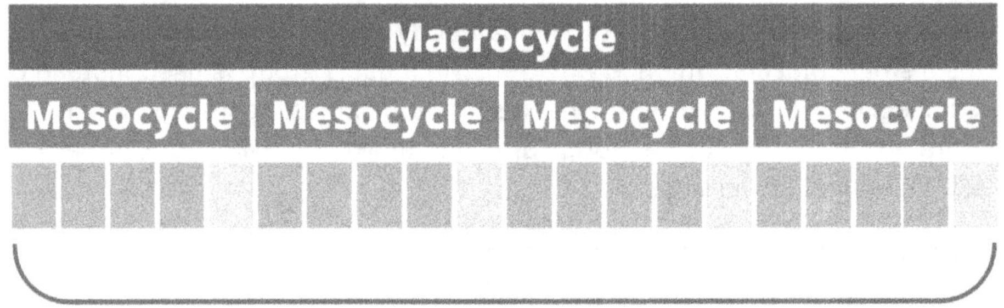

Microcycles

For simplicity, for the rest of this book a microcycle will be one week, the standard length as it is generally the easiest timeframe to schedule around.

<u>Deloads:</u>

A deload period (notated by the paler blocks) is a programmed period of recovery, roughly the length of a single microcycle, where training volume is greatly reduced. This can be done by reducing the load for each exercise (usually by about 50%), reducing the number of sets for each exercise (usually by about 50%), or a combination of both methods. In either case, the rep ranges shouldn't change, which means that RPE (page 23) is much lower, and in fact too low to induce a hypertrophic stimulus.

The purpose of the a deload week is to allow for the essential recovery of muscles, systemic fatigue and perhaps most importantly, joints and connective tissues, which take longer to recover than muscular fatigue. By still training with light volume however, the neurological movement patterns are still getting trained, which promote strength.

Training without deload weeks would not only gradually cause performance to decline as fatigue accumulates but would also increase the risk of injury. It may seem that there is a sweet spot of volume whereby deloads are unnecessary. It is possible to train this way however it would be suboptimal as the intensity and volume would have to be reduced considerably to make this a sustainable approach – it's much better to train with high effort and high volumes with regular deloads than to consistently train with medium effort. Deloads should be taken if you believe you are overtraining.

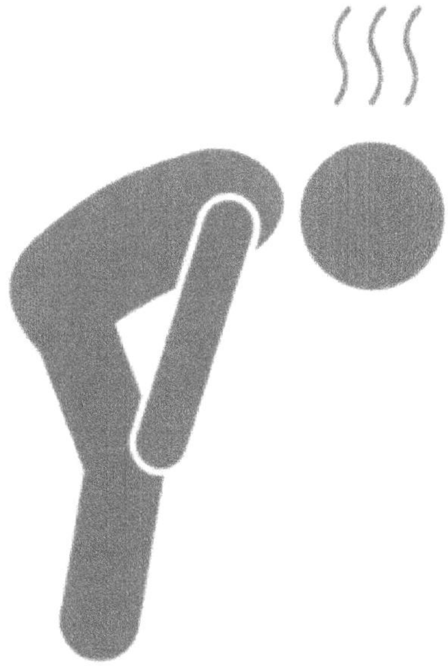

<u>Training variables</u>

Although the training variables are very dependent on each other, here is a pyramid showing a general hierarchy:

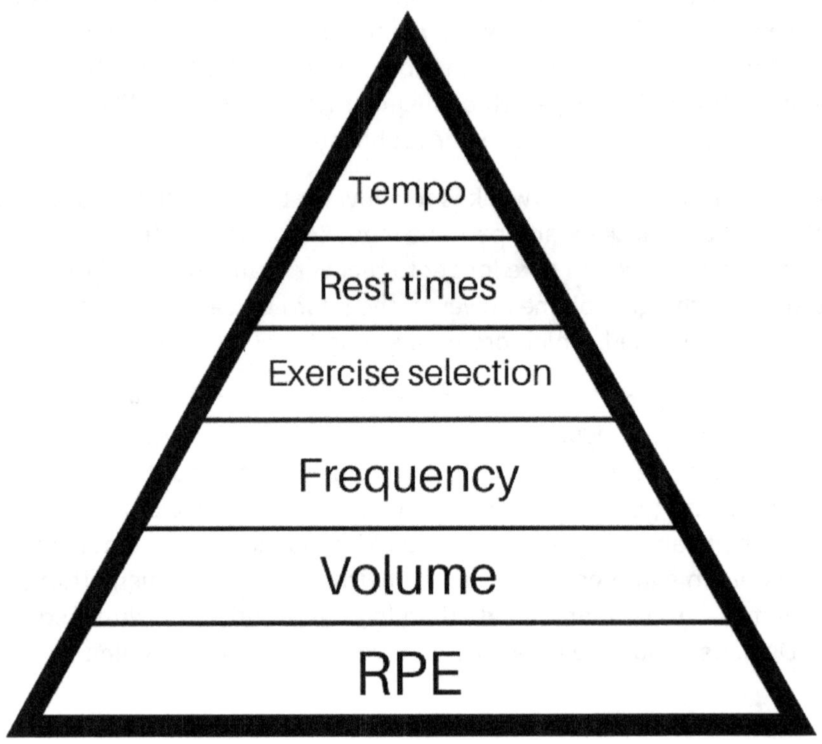

RPE/RIR:

The first training variable that must be considered is the effort of workouts. Given as a rating out of 10, rate of perceived exertion (RPE) refers to how close to failure a set is taken; eg. RPE 9 refers to a set taken to 1 rep away from failure. Oppositely, reps in reserve (RIR) refers to the number of reps away from technical failure a set is taken to; eg. RIR 2 refers to a set taken to 2 reps from failure. Beginners tend to overestimate how close to failure they train so once comfortable performing a exercises safely, it is a good idea to take a single set of each to true failure with a given load to test this. Online calculators can be used to calculate a 1RM and the load to use for a given number or reps.

There is a threshold at which you must train beyond to induce hypertrophic stimulus. The closer to failure you train, the greater the stimulus, but the greater the fatigue too. The graph below shows a simplified relationship between stimulus and fatigue at different RPEs, which will differ between muscle groups and individuals.

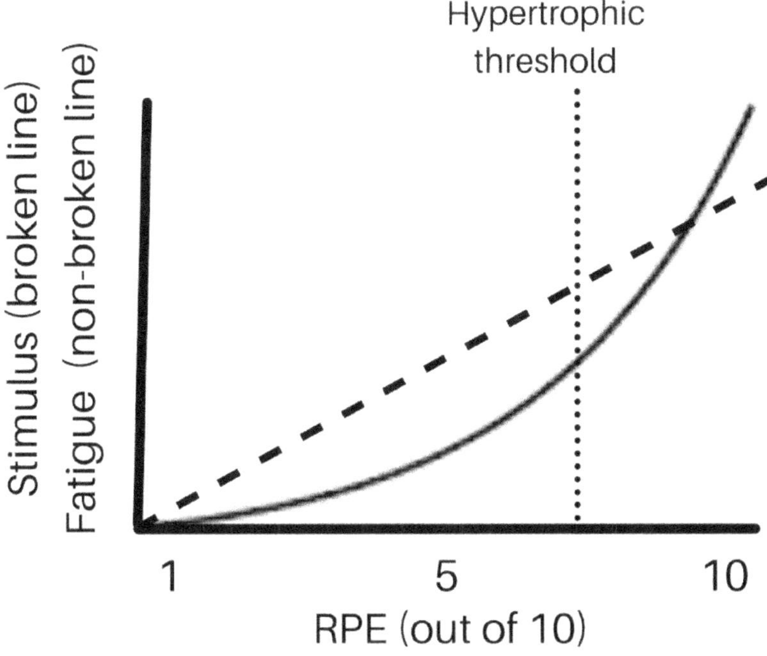

From this we can see that always training to failure frequently is not sustainable. It is better to train to RPE 8/9 (1/2 RIR) and train more frequently. The additional gains made from training all the way to failure as opposed to 1/2 RIR is generally not worth the extra fatigue it induces, which will comprise performance of upcoming sets. Furthermore, rest times both between sets and between exercises would have to be increased to accommodate for the extra recovery needed. Volume will be particularly compromised when training to failure in the strength rep range (page 26) which is the most fatiguing. The risk of injury is also much higher when training for closer to failure, so instead of always maxing out the pump, just remember the phrase "stimulate, not annihilate".

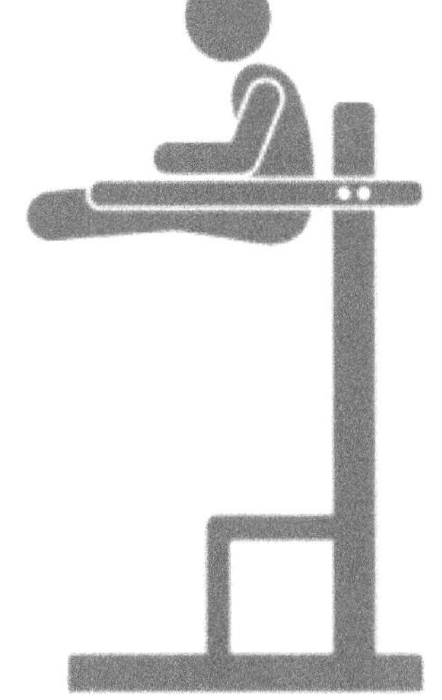

<u>Variation of RPE:</u>

As we must train within about 2 reps shy of failure to induce the necessary stimulus, RPE has limited capacity for progressive overload. It can increase from 8 to 10 throughout the mesocycle as although higher RPE also induces more fatigue, this extra fatigue is worth the extra stimulus during the last week of a mesocycle as a recovery deload week follows, allowing the fatigue to dissipate. As a guide, train closer to failure the closer you are to deloading. There are some exceptions to this however:

1) Compound exercises carry high risk of injury when performed at RPE 9/10. All beginners should have the necessary precautions (eg. a spotter) in place if attempting these lifts at these RPEs. It is acceptable to train at RPE 9 for compounds in the last week before deloading, rather than 10.

2) Isolations don't carry as much fatigue and so can be trained much closer to failure. 0/1 RIR is a good target for isolation exercises. The last set of the last exercise of a muscle group in a workout can go all the way to failure if it is an isolation movement.

3) For beginners, exercise form will likely break down the closer to failure they train. So, for absolute beginners, start with about RPE 7 until comfortable performing the exercises, so as to not engrain bad movement patterns when grinding out bad reps at the end of a set.

It is important not to progress RPE too fast, which is tempting to do, as this will lead to overtraining. The best way to ensure that RPE is not being over programmed is by autoregulating. This essentially means training with the RPE that you feel you can handle on the day. This cannot be an excuse for laziness – you should still stick to your programme as closely as possible but autoregulating is an acceptable means of monitoring when to push closer to failure for each exercise, remembering that the RPE should only increase throughout the mesocycle for each exercise.

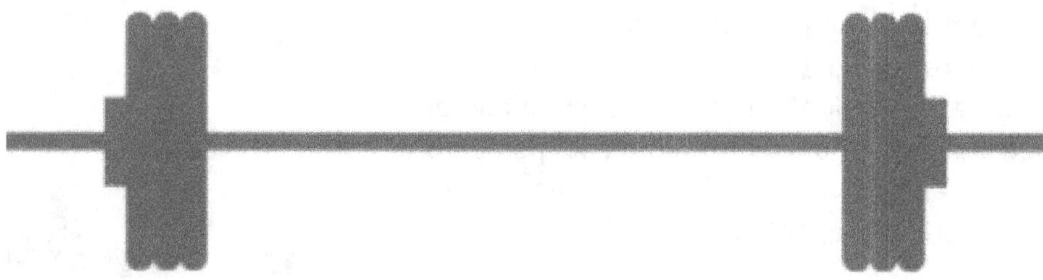

Volume:

The first aspects of volume to consider are the numbers of reps per set and load, which are inversely proportionate to each other. Lifting heavier will mean less reps, for the same RPE. The question of whether to lift heavy with low reps or lift light with heavy reps depends on your goal. The rep range spectrum below shows that 0-5 reps is optimal for strength, 6-12 is optimal for hypertrophy, and 13+ is optimal for endurance, assuming a training effort of at least RPE 8. There is crossover between rep ranges.

Number of reps in a set
(training within at least 3 reps of failure)

1 2 3 4 5 6 7 8 9 10 11 12 13 14 15 16 17 18 19 20

Strength	Hypertrophy	Muscular endurance
>80% 1RM	60%-85% 1RM	<70% 1RM

Load used for set

Different muscle types also respond better to different rep ranges due to their muscle fibres. Type I, "slow twitch" fibres are more resistant to endurance and so benefit more from higher rep ranges. Type II "fast twitch" fibres are more powerful and less fatigue resistant so respond better to lower rep ranges. Different muscle groups will contain different ratios of these fibres and so the rep ranges for exercises should reflect this (although not taken to the extreme); eg. use higher end of hypertrophy rep range for calves (mostly type I) and lower range for chest (mostly type II). As 6-12 is still a fairly big range, your programme should reflect a more constricted rep range to work in; eg. 5-8 reps or 8-12 reps. A range should still be used rather than a single target as the number of reps will likely decrease by 1 or 2 between sets of the same exercise, as the target muscle fatigues. The load can be reduced if the reps fall out of the programmed rep range, although this should be done sparingly as it will reduce volume.

Once the rep range and therefore load has been determined, the number of sets will determine the weekly volume. As the graph below shows, training with higher volumes will induce greater stimulus, and therefore more hypertrophic adaptations to occur. This is true up to a point where the fatigue that is also induced outweighs the stimulus and so increasing volume after this point becomes less effective.

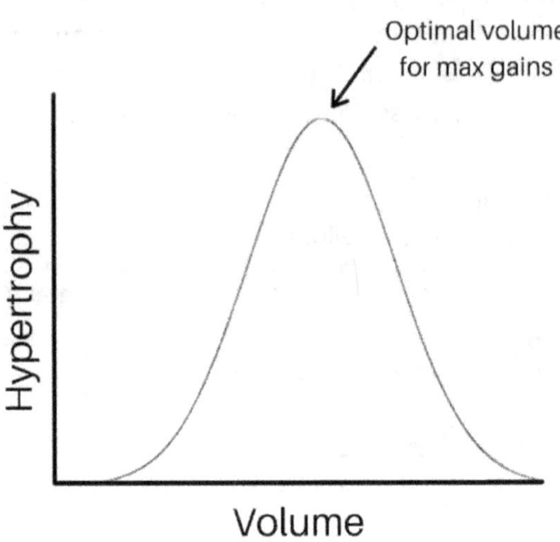

The x-axis could be labelled "number of sets", as rep range and load will be constant (until strength adaptations occur).

At the peak, no more volume can be added without the fatigue becoming so high that full recovery doesn't occur – overtraining. Volume must be managed at every scope for optimal gains.

Volume must be considered carefully, especially by beginners who will not know their optimal weekly volume. Beginners should begin with low volume (especially on big compounds), as the novelty of training will provide sufficient stimulus. By starting light, this will also allow beginners to focus on technique. There should be at least 3 sets for each exercise to produce enough stimulus. Different muscle groups will need a different number of weekly sets which is highly individual and dependant on the other training variables. Remembering that compound movements target multiple muscle groups, a general guide is to have 10-20 weekly sets for each muscle group. Beginners will tend to be at the bottom of this range.

Volume should also be considered holistically. Excessive collective volume would cause too much systemic fatigue.

<u>Variation of volume:</u>

Even for hypertrophy training, utilising the strength and endurance rep ranges is beneficial. By getting stronger from training in the 0-5 rep range, you will be able to cope with higher loads which will mean more volume. Endurance training will increase your rep capacity during sets which also will increase volume. Therefore, it is recommended to train in the hypertrophic rep range about 70-80% of the time and utilise the strength and endurance rep ranges for the rest of your training. This should be done periodically and can be done any level of scope cycle: Rep ranges could vary between exercises of the same muscle group within a workout, between workouts or between mesocycles. Varying between mesocycles is preferable, as it will allow you to focus on progressive overload for a given rep range for a several weeks.

It is generally agreed that the progression of volume is the most influential overloading factor for hypertrophy. Rep ranges are determined by your specific goal and so cannot be continually increased. The number of sets can be increased throughout the mesocycle, however this has limited application as eventually, workouts would become too time-consuming and fatiguing, which would reduce performance and stimulate endurance rather than hypertrophy. As hypertrophy training has carry over with strength training (as seen in the rep ranges chart), the best way to progressively overload volume is to increase load, as you get stronger.

A good way to do this is to start at the lower limit your rep range, work up to the upper limit, increase the load so that you are back at the bottom of the rep range and then repeat this cycle. Increasing the number of sets of some exercises over the course of the mesocycle can also be beneficial, but most of the volume overload should come from increasing load. **This is the fundamental principle of hypertrophy training.** There are other ways of progressing volume and as long as you stay within the programmed rep range and RPE, the method of progression doesn't matter too much.

The progression in load each workout needless be excessive - regular, incremental progress is the way to go. Imagine the progress over the course of one year from adding 1/2kg to each of your compound lifts each week. Beginners adapt quickly and so should be able to increase load frequently. Volume should be progressed so that, like RPE, it is high at the end of a mesocycle. The extra stimulus is worth the fatigue in the last microcycle as the deload that come after it allows for recovery of fatigue.

Frequency:

Frequency simply refers to how the volume for each muscle group is distributed over the week. Training with higher frequency provides more opportunity for protein synthesis. Different muscles recover at different rates but generally, protein synthesis usually lasts about 2-3 days (when trained at high effort), so it would be optimal to train every muscle every 2/3 days. Distributing the volume for each muscle group over the week would optimise performance - training excessive volume for a muscle group in a single workout would mean that the last few sets or even exercises are performed sub-optimally (less reps or lighter load, therefore less volumes) due to the muscular fatigue accumulated throughout the workout. For the same volume, training a muscle group twice a week is more beneficial than training it only once, but there is no strong evidence that proves three times is better than two. Therefore, it would be a good idea to train all muscle groups at least twice a week, and the smaller ones thrice (as they can recover faster). By splitting up the volume for each muscle group across the week, performance is consistent.

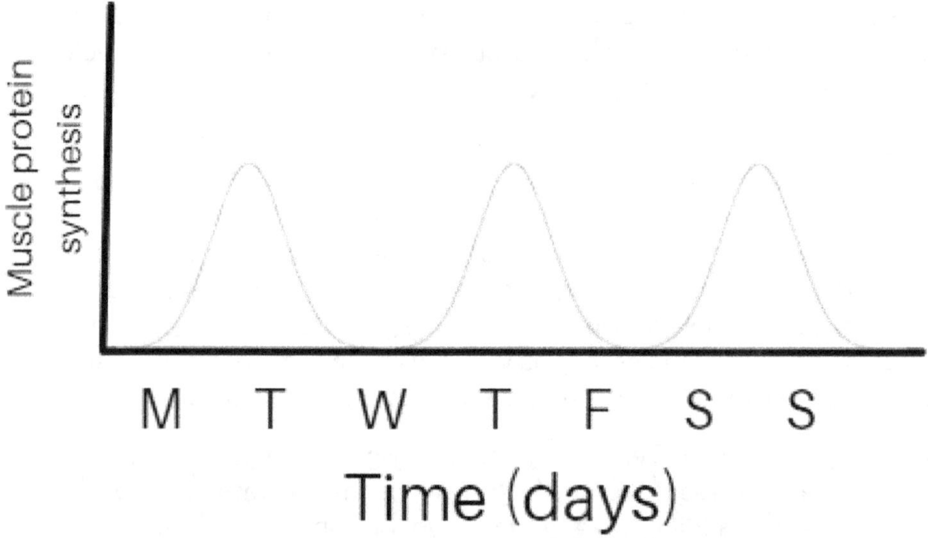

Splitting 9 sets for a muscle group into 3 sets on Monday, Wednesday, and Friday creates 3 spikes in muscle protein synthesis (remembering that protein synthesis occurs during the rest after the workout).

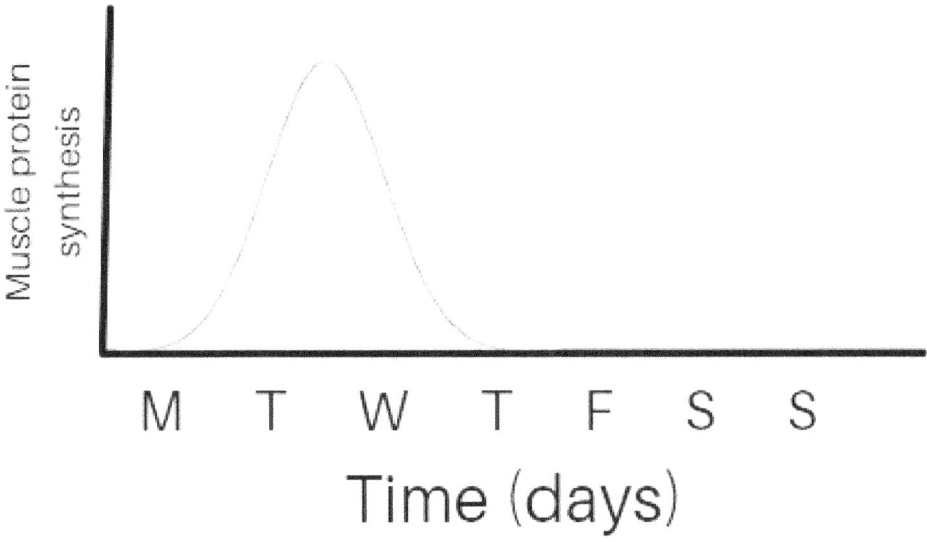

Training all 9 sets on Monday doesn't take advantage of higher frequency training. The stimulus would be higher during Monday's workout, however as this only causes one period of protein synthesis, it would result in less hypertrophy by the end of the week in comparison to the first example.

As smaller muscle groups can recover faster, they can be trained at higher frequencies – up to 4/5 times a week dependant on volume.

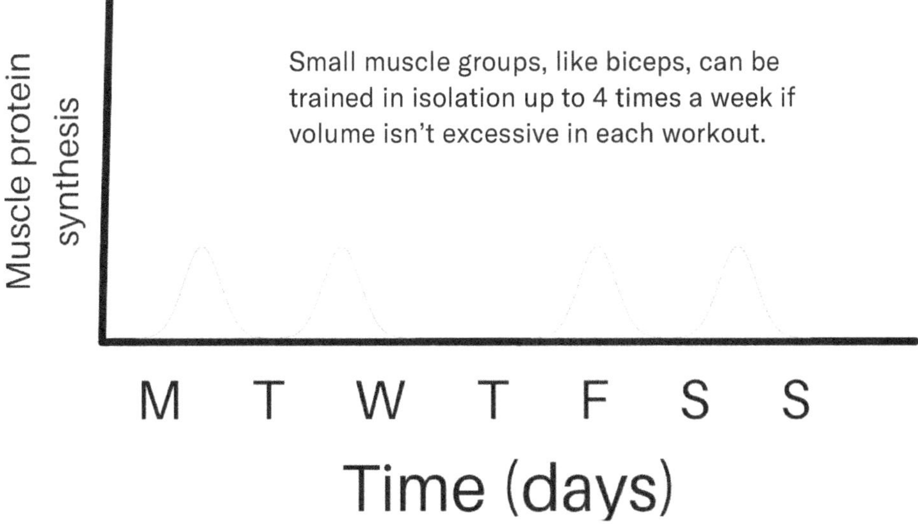

This is, however, complicated by the fact that compound movements train multiple muscle groups in different proportions. It is impossible to quote the relative stimulation various muscle groups acquire in compound exercises, but as a guide, assume that the non-dominant muscle groups get half the stimulation they would if they were trained in isolation; eg. when performing 4 sets of pull ups, assume biceps (non-dominant muscle group) receive half the volume and frequency (2 sets), but the back (dominant) receives the full volume and frequency (4 sets). This is exemplified on page 48.

Delayed onset muscle soreness (DOMS), is reduced when training at higher frequencies. Various training splits (part 4) distribute volume differently.

<u>Variation of frequency:</u>

Weekly frequency should be inversely proportionate to workout volume and so should not be increased for progressive overload but should be varied for novelty. Muscle groups should be trained 2-4 times a week and the frequency of each can be varied between mesocycles, or every few mesocycles.

Eg. Mesocycles 1 and 2:

Train 2x /week:	Train 3x / week:
Chest	Back
Triceps	Traps
Abs	Biceps
Shoulders	
Quads	
Glutes	
Hamstrings	
Calves	

Mesocycles 3 and 4:

2x / week:	3x / week:
Back	Chest
Traps	Triceps
Biceps	Abs
Shoulders	
Quads	
Glutes	
Hamstrings	
Calves	

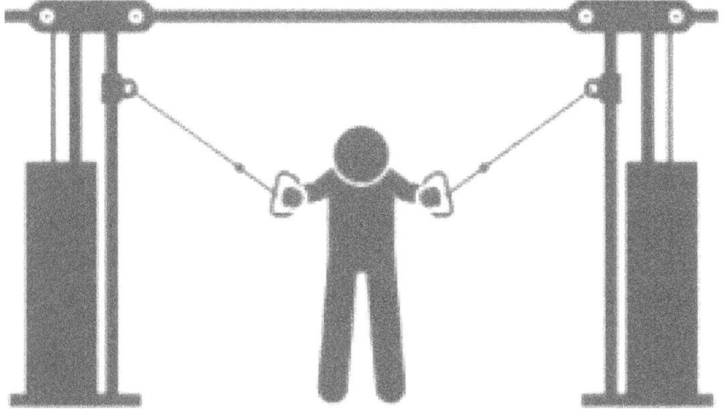

Exercise selection:

Exercise selection is the next most important consideration for a training programme. When choosing the specific exercises, the following should be considered:

1) Trainees should always consider the importance of building a balanced physique. Exclusively training "beach muscles" like arms and chest whilst neglecting legs and back will result in poor posture and injuries in the long term. As a guide, include as roughly as many pushing movements as pulling movements - longevity must at the forefront of programme design.

2) Gym machines like multigyms and cables tend to focus on isolation exercises and can be used where necessary, but most movements should be free weight exercises which provide the additional benefit of working stabiliser muscles. Beginners should focus mainly on compound movements that can be divided into the following categories:

   Horizontal push

   Horizontal pull

   Vertical push

   Vertical pull

   Leg exercises (knee flexion and hip extension)

   Of course, weights are always lifted upwards, against gravity; the horizontal plane is relative to the body - when lying down for bench press, the weight is being push upwards, but horizontal to the body and so is a horizontal push exercise.

3) Compound exercises are easier to overload and so more efficient. Barbells will be able to lift more weight than the combined load of dumbbells for the same exercise due to stability. Isolation exercises should function as accessory movements for these big lifts.

4) Exercises can be anything that provide a stimulus however some are better than others. The best exercises are ones which provide the most stimulus to the target muscle, but least fatigue. Deadlifts are a popular lift and whilst they stimulate most muscles in the body, the fatigue it carries is one of the highest of any lift.

5) Individuals should select exercises where the target muscle is felt working and is the limiting factor for every set - there is little point performing bicep curls if the fatigue/burn in the forearms prevents the biceps from getting close enough to failure to induce a hypertrophic stimulus. Depending on the RPE for the exercise, the local fatigue in the biceps should be the only thing preventing more reps in every set of bicep curls, not cardio fatigue, or local fatigue of another muscle group. For compound lifts, the limiting factor should be the local fatigue of the dominant muscle group; eg. quads during squats.

<u>Variation for exercise selection:</u>

To train each muscle group, there of course needs to be a variety of exercises throughout the week. For each muscle group, 2-3 exercises are plenty. Exercises should be consistent week to week, and only varied each mesocycle slightly, if at all. Changing as often as each week would prevent progressive overload over the course of the mesocycle but never varying exercises would eventually lead to stale training, where the body is too comfortable with the exercises and so won't respond much to the stimulus. When choosing different exercises for the same muscle group, sometimes it is good to target different sub-groups of the muscle; eg. when choosing two exercises for the chest, choose one that focusses on the upper chest and one that focusses on the mid chest. This type of variation could also be applied between mesocycles; eg. focus on mid chest for one or two mesocycles, and then upper chest for the next one or two mesocycles. Beginners shouldn't need this kind of exercise variation for a while and should stick to the basic variations of exercises; eg. flat bench press. These big compound movements should also not be varied often as they are the easiest to overload with volume and most resistant to staleness.

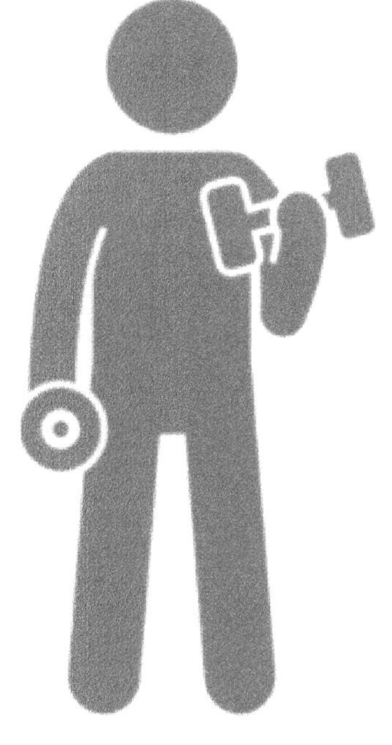

All exercises must be performed with correct form. Exercise execution is covered in part 5.

Rest times:

Rest times are required between sets, between workouts (rest days) and between mesocycles (deloads). Rest times between sets do not need to be timed, however there should be enough rest to ensure that the upcoming set provides a good stimulus to the target muscle. This means enough rest to hit the programmed rep range in the upcoming set and ensure that the target muscle is the limiting factor preventing performance of more reps. This means enough rest to ensure that nor cardio or fatigue of a non-targeted muscle group limits the number of reps in the upcoming set.

Number of reps in a set
(training within at least 3 reps of failure)

1 2 3 4 5 6 7 8 9 10 11 12 13 14 15 16 17 18 19 20

Strength	Hypertrophy	Muscular endurance
>3 minutes	1-3 minutes	<1 minute

Rest time between sets

When training in the strength rep range, rest times will need to be longer and when training for endurance, rest times should be shorter. Here is a spectrum of approximate rest times for each rep range, again assuming that effort is at least RPE 8.

Too little rest will reduce the number of reps on the upcoming set and too much rest is simply unnecessary. Isolation exercises and exercises for smaller muscle groups will require less rest both between sets and between workouts than larger muscle groups. Rest times do not need to be varied.

Phases and tempo

There are four phases to dynamic exercises:

1) The concentric phase where a muscle contracts to move a weight against gravity; eg. the arm raise in lateral raise.

2) The isometric phase where a muscle maintains contraction, staying the same length, to keep a weight from falling under the influence of gravity; eg. the top hold of a lateral raise.

3) The eccentric phase where a muscle gradually relaxes to lower a weight; eg. the arm lowering in a lateral raise.

4) The resting phase where the target muscle is relaxed; eg. the bottom part of a lateral raise (no tension).

There is some contention as to whether loaded stretching (the resting phase) induces hypertrophic stimulus, but the first three phases definitely do, so it is important utilise all phases by controlling the weight all through the movement, especially during the eccentric phase where it is tempting to let the weight fall. Controlled reps also reduce the risk of injury, particularly during heavy weight compounds.

Tempo (or cadence) refers to the relative time spent in each phase of the movement; eg. a 2-0-2-1 would refer to a 2 second eccentric, 0 second rest, 2 second concentric, and 1 second isometric. The tempo and number of reps in a set determine the time under tension for which a muscle is put through. For a given load, higher time under tension will provide more stimulus. Tempo is a very minor variable and does not need to be over-considered; a split-second squeeze at the top and split-second stretch at the bottom is recommended to discourage bouncing and using momentum to cheat reps. As longs as the tempo is roughly consistent between reps and all phases are controlled, tempo does not need to be varied.

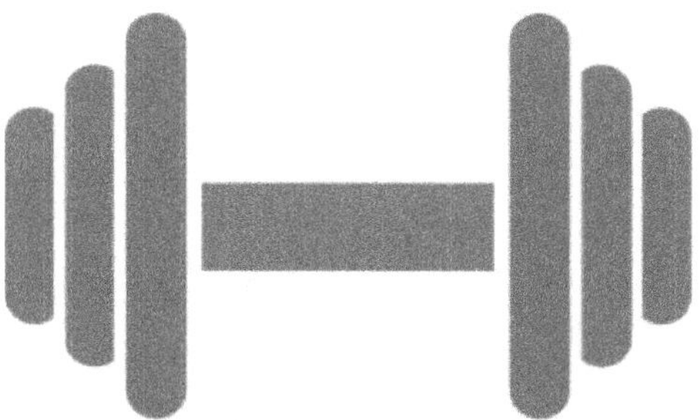

Summary of how and when to vary training variables:

Variable	How to vary	When to vary
RIR	Train at RPE 8 or higher (absolute beginners can start at RPE 7) This can increase to 9 or 10 RPE	Throughout mesocycle Last week of mesocycle should be at least RPE 9, isolations should be RPE 10
Volume	Work upwards through rep range then increase load Can also add sets in moderation	Increase load as often as possible Increase sets throughout mesocycle (optional)
Frequency	Vary which muscle groups are trained at higher frequencies	Between weeks, or between mesocycles / every few mesocycles (recommended)
Exercise Selection	Change exercises for each muscle group	Strictly between mesocycles or every few mesocycles
Rest time	Varying frequency of muscle groups automatically change the rest times between workouts Rest times between sets do not need to be varied	/
Tempo	Tempo does not need to be varied	/

The training variables can also be manipulated to overcome plateaus in training:

Eg. train using different rep ranges

Eg. train with a different frequency

Eg. change exercises

Eg. reduce tempo to create more time under tension

Part 4: Programme Design

Training splits

There are many ways to distribute exercises over the week, but a beginner should base their programme on one of the following training splits.

Split name	Eg. split	Advantages	Disadvantages
Full body	M – full body T – rest W – full body T – rest F – full body S – rest S - rest	High frequency so frequent overload Learn movement patterns quickly	Little volume per muscle group per workout Cannot sustainably train consecutive days
Upper lower	M – upper body T – rest W – lower body T – rest F – upper body S – lower body S - rest	2x week is a good frequency Train related muscle groups	Upper body generally requires more exercises so workouts may not be consistent in number of exercises
Push pull (includes legs)	M – push T – rest W – pull T – rest F – push S – pull S - rest	2x week is a good frequency Train related muscle groups each workout	Do not train antagonistic muscle groups in the same workout
Push pull legs (push and pull only for upper body)	M – push T – pull W – legs T – rest F – push S – pull S - legs	Can train back to back days as training different muscle groups	Only 1 rest day which may be unsustainable for some Alternative of once each a week is low fequency
Bro split (each muscle group trained on a different day)	M – Arms T – Chest W – Back T – Rest F – Legs S – Shoulders/abs S - rest	Each muscle group has 7 days to recover (although this is more than necessary)	Very low frequency Performance will decrease throughout workout as muscles fatigue

The number of training days a week for each can be varied, but examples of how the different workouts are distributed over the week are given. Training days could be split over a 2 week period:

Eg. a push pull split could be rearranged to form a two-week cycle:

M – Push	M - Pull
T – Pull	T - Push
W – Rest	W – Rest
T – Push	T - Pull
F – Pull	F - Push
S – Push	S - Pull
S – Rest	S – Rest

.

It is recommended that beginners start with a full body routine and maintain this training split for at least 2/3 mesocycles. This is because it trains few exercises, allowing the beginner to become proficient at them and allowing them to be overloaded frequently. For an absolute beginner, there is no need to overcomplicate the training programme as the novelty of training will provide sufficient stimulation without the need for excessive manipulation of the training variables. The most effective programme for a beginner will be a simple one. After several mesocycles of a full body routine, other splits can be employed to vary training. Whist this is not essential, it will keep training enjoyable.

After utilising full body splits for some time, the beginner should progress to a two-part split routine such as an upper/lower split or a push/pull split for variation. Full body splits can be recycled later if desired. Bro splits should generally be avoided as the lack of frequency makes them much weaker than the other splits.

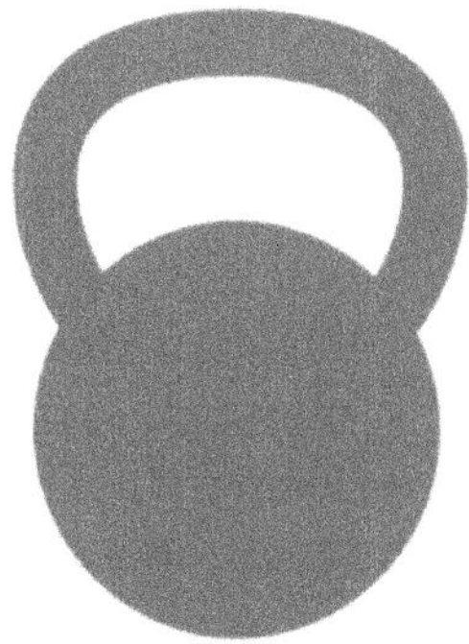

Guidelines for designing your programme

1) Your programme should be based around a microcycle, usually a single week. Decide how many days a week you want to work out, based on your lifestyle; a more active lifestyle will mean less capacity for training in the gym and so fewer days (or shorter workouts).

2) Decide on the split to use as a foundation – they can be modified with some creativity. The split can be a weekly/biweekly cycle or anything in between. For absolute beginners, a 3-times a week full body split is often best.

3) The week of training should include exercises that train the following movements at least twice a week:

    A horizontal push
    A horizontal pull
    A vertical push
    A vertical pull
    2 leg exercises – 1 knee extension exercise and 1 hip flexion exercise

This could be the same or different exercises for each category. Each workout should start with 2/3 compound movements, followed by 2/3 isolation movements. The compound exercises should generally be ordered primary (heavy exercises that target big muscles) followed by secondary (exercises that target smaller muscle groups). There should be at least as many primary and secondary exercises combined as isolation exercises for each workout.

It is acceptable to have 1/2 isolations that do not align with the split but are implemented to optimise frequency; eg. Training abs 3 times a week utilises frequency and so implementing them into a push day (as well as two pull days of a push pull split), they can be targeted 3 times a week. A push day of a push pull split could be:

    Squats   - compound (primary)
    Bench press   - compound (primary)
    Overhead press   - compound (secondary)
    Skull crushers   - isolation (accessory)
    Leg raises   - isolation (accessory), not a push exercise,
                          but can still be implemented into push day if
                          wanting to train abs at a high frequency

4) The compound exercises should be mostly free weight lifts.

5) There should be a ratio of about 2:1 upper body to lower body exercises as there are more planes of motion in the upper body to train.

6) Bigger muscle groups will take longer to recover and so should be spread out more across the week than smaller muscle groups. Performing heavy squats 2 days in a row would be unwise as the quads will be recovering during the second workout, resulting sub-optimal performance.

7) A huge selection of exercises is unnecessary – it's better to become proficient at fewer exercises. There should be about 5/6 exercises per workout, with each workout lasting 45-90 minutes. This will ensure that you are not too fatigued, and muscles are still being stimulated efficiently at the end of the workout.

8) Programme roughly as many pushing movements as pulling movements for a balanced physique. An exception to this is that anterior deltoids needless be trained in isolation as they receive a lot of stimulus from the various pushing movements such as bench press and overhead press. The rear deltoids can be trained in isolation, particularly if a programme favours pushing over pulling.

9) It is up to the individual whether they want to train forearms and calves in isolation. Forearms will receive stimulus from heaving compound pulls such as deadlift and pull ups but can be targeted in isolation too. Calves are often regarded as the hardest muscle to grow, and beginners may want to diverge their efforts to the rest of the body for the first year of training.

10) Cardio can be scheduled into workouts, depending on lifestyle factors and goals. For a sedentary individual, light/medium intensity runs on rest days can be beneficial to weightlifting and general health. If wanting to train cardio on workout days, it should be placed after the workout. This should, however, be avoided on days that train legs.

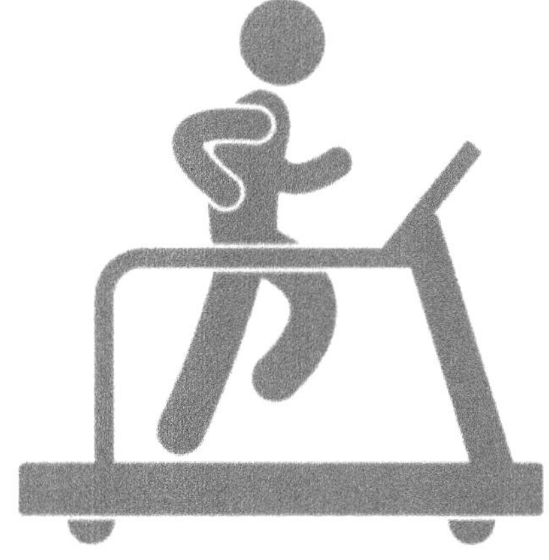

Example split

Here is an example of a 3-times a week full body split. All compounds will be trained for 4 sets, and all isolations for 3:

Bold: Compound exercise

Underlined: Standard primary exercise

DL: Deadlift

OHP: Overhead press

BB: Barbell

M	T	W	T	F	S	S
BB bench press	Rest	**DL**	Rest	**BB OHP**	Rest	Rest (Light run)
BB back squat		**BB OHP**		**BB back squat**		
Pull ups		**BB row**		**BB bench press**		
Hamstring curls		Face pulls		**BB row**		
Leg raises		Hamstring curls		Leg raises		
Standing calf raises		Standing calf raises		Face pulls		

<u>Why this programme works:</u>

1) It is built around 6 different compound movements covering the 4 upper body planes of motion as well as legs:

   Bench – horizontal push
   OHP – vertical push
   Row – horizontal pull
   Pull up – vertical pull
   DL – Hip extension
   Squat – Knee flexion

2) The compound exercises are placed before the isolations as they are more fatiguing. There are also at least 3 compounds per workout and the number of isolation movements doesn't exceed this.

   Although keeping compound before isolations, same or similar exercises are in different positions on different days; eg. hamstring curls occur once as the fourth exercise and once as the fifth to vary which muscle group is trained when more fatigued. This also applies to the compound exercises –bench press is first on Monday, but third on Friday. This isn't compulsory; the standard primary movements could consistently be placed before the secondary ones.

   In this example, calves are trained last on both days as they are not affected but any of the previous exercises (apart from systemic fatigue) and are the least fatiguing exercise to perform.

3) Every muscle group is trained at least twice a week, with the smaller ones (anterior and rear deltoids) trained more frequently. (Triceps are also trained frequently but this is fine as they are never trained in isolation). Muscle groups have ample time to recover, with the larger group needing up to 48 hours and the smaller ones needing slightly less.

4) 5-6 exercises per workout means that with 3/4 sets per exercise, the workout will last between 45 and 90 minutes.

5) The most intense day (Friday, as it contains 4 compound exercises) has the most rest after it (2 days). This is a small, but purposeful detail.

The following table shows the weekly frequency (hitting the same muscle group twice in one workout counts as 1) and number of sets for each muscle group for this programme

Muscle group	Exercise	Weekly frequency	Weekly number of sets (non-dominant muscle groups of compound exercises count as half)
Chest	Bench press (horizontal push)	2	8
Back in vertical plane	Pull ups DL (vertical pulls)	2	8
Back in horizontal plane	Row (horizontal pull)	2	8
Spinal erectors	DL, squats	3	8 (counting squats as half)
Traps	DL, face pulls	2	8 (counting DL as half)
Anterior deltoid	Bench press, OHP (vertical push)	3	8 (counting bench press and OHP as half)
Medial deltoid	OHP	2	8
Rear deltoid	Pull ups, face pulls, rows	3	12 (counting pull ups and rows as half)
Biceps	Pull ups, rows	3	6 (counting pull ups and rows as half)
Triceps	Bench press, OHP	3	8 (counting bench press and OHP as half)
Abs	Leg raises	2	6
Quads	Squats, DL	3	10 (counting DL as half)
Glutes	Squats, DL	3	8 (counting squats as half)
Hamstrings	Curls	2	6
Forearms	Pull ups, DL, rows	3	8 (counting pull ups, DL and rows as half)
Calves	Raises	2	6

It's hard for a beginner to gauge how much volume is optimal foreach muscle group, but these weekly volumes are a good guide. The volume could be increased by adding more sets for some exercises if necessary. Alternatively, if you wanted to emphasis one muscle group for a mesocycle or two, the programme could be modified; eg. for bicep focus, substitute bicep curls for calf training on Monday and Wednesday and implement calve raises in a later mesocycle.

<u>Gym myths</u>:

Many beginners think that doing light ab work such as a timed sit up routine at the end of every workout, or even every day, will increase abdominal definition. Although abs are a small muscle group which can be trained frequently, they still require progressive overload and recovery in order to grow, so training abs regularly is good as long as it is overloaded each time. By never progressing the number of reps, sets or load, overload is not being progressed and so gains will plateau.

Many people also believe that ab exercises will exclusively reduce fat around the abdominal area. During fat loss, fat is reduced from all over the body and so performing specific exercises that target specific body parts will not "spot reduce" fat in that area. Genetics play a big role in body fat distribution.

Ab definition requires a body fat percentage of about 15% for men and about 20% for women. Extreme leanness is unhealthy and should not be maintained for long periods of time.

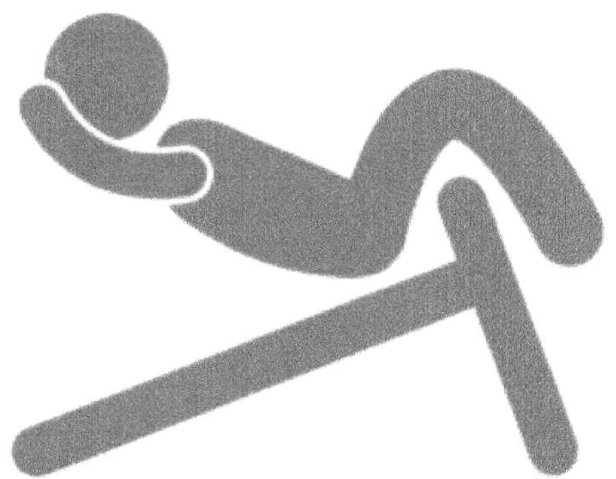

Summary

Your first programme may not be perfect; you can adapt it whilst you discover what works well for you. Getting 80% right is a great start, so focus on the more important factors like longevity, specificity and progressive overload. Finer details should be considered afterwards.

Combining everything, here is a general hierarchy pyramid of considerations for a training programme, all of which should be tailored to your specific goal:

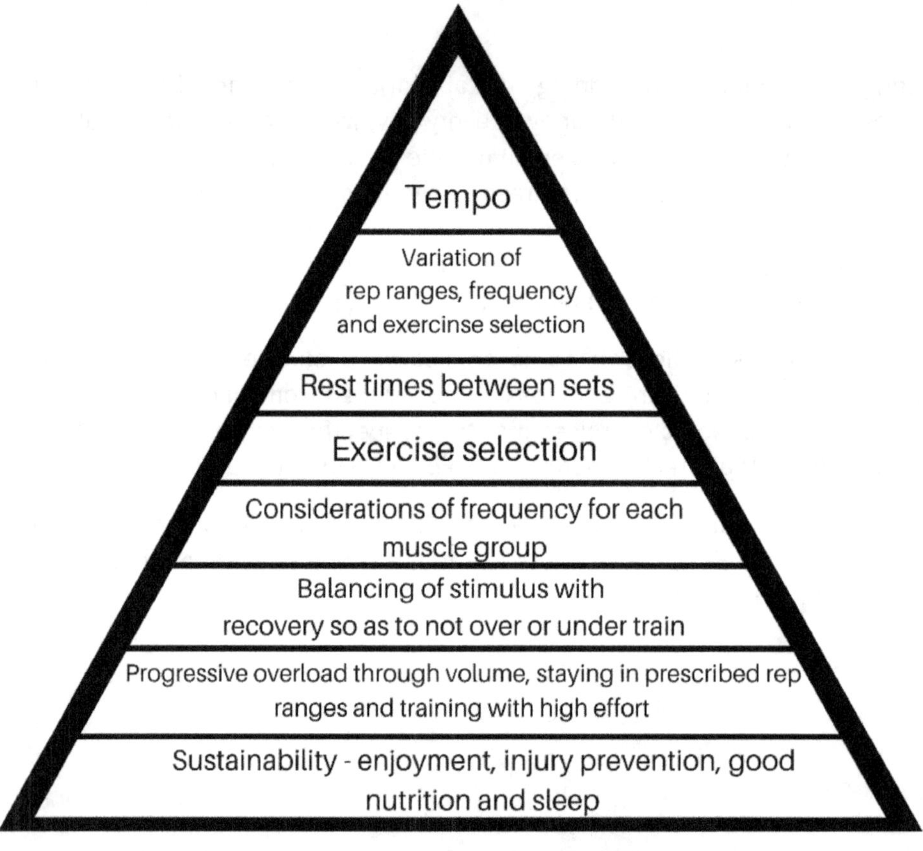

Build a strong foundation in both your programme and training and focus on the micro details later - most of your results will come from the foundations.

Off-days happen for every athlete. You should only re-evaluate your programme if you incur consistent bad days, which most likely will be due to overprogrammed volume - overtraining. Mistakes are inevitable and, in fact, a key part of learning so don't be put off from making them.

Part 5: Practical Advice

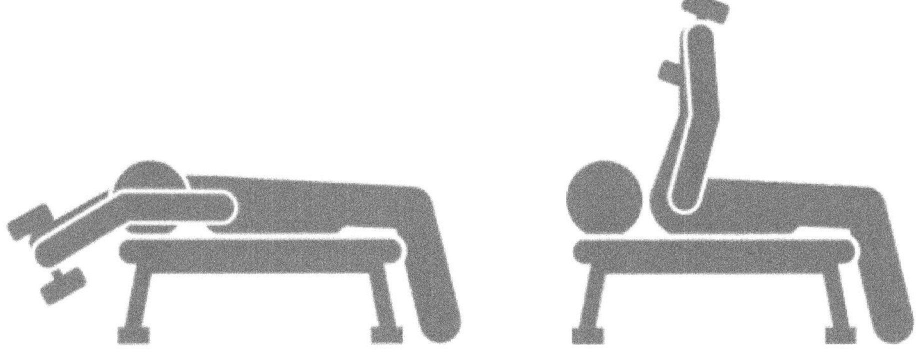

Tracking progress

Logging workouts to track progress is often overlooked by beginners but is the best way to ensure exercises are being overloaded. Overload doesn't need to happen every time you train the same exercise but at least each week is good. To track progress, log the sets, reps, and load for every exercise as a minimum, which should be improved in some way next time round. A template for a single workout could look like this:

Training day 1, week 1	Target rep range	Reps in each set	Load (kg)	RIR	Approximate rest time between sets (min)	Approximate tempo (sec)	Additional notes, eg. form cues
Exercise A	5-8	7,6,5,5	V	2	3	2,0,1,0	
Exercise B	5-8	8,8,7	W	2	2.5	1,0,1,0	
Exercise C	8-10	10,9,9	X	2	2.5	1,0,1,1	
Exercise D	8-10	9,9,8,8	Y	1	1	2,1,2,1	
Exercise E	10-12	12,12,11	Z	1	1	2,1,2,1	

Although the exercises aren't disclaimed here, they should be logged in the order that they are performed. The initial compounds (**bold**) will require longer rest times due to heavier loads, as shown.

Reps may sometimes decrease by 1/2 between sets which is fine, as long as they stay within the prescribed rep range.

The additional column allows you to note useful form cues which will encourage good form; eg. pull with elbows during pull ups (rather than hands).

The rest time and tempo columns could be omitted as they will generally stay constant week to week. The same could be said for RIR, but it is good practice for beginners to write this down to gauge how much effort they are putting into their workouts. The next time this workout is performed, the volume should be increased, even if only slightly. This could be by lifting heavier weights and performing the same number of reps, performing more reps with the same weight, or performing more reps with a heavier weight.

The following week may look like this:

Training day 1, week 2	Target rep range	Reps in each set	Load (kg)	RIR	Approximate rest time between sets (min)	Approximate tempo (s)	Additional notes eg. form cues
Exercise A	5-8	8,7,6,5	V	2	3	2,0,1,0	
Exercise B	5-8	7,7,7	W+2	2	2.5	1,0,1,0	
Exercise C	8-10	10,9,9	X+2	2	2	1,0,1,1	
Exercise D	8-10	9,9,9,9	Y	1	1	2,1,2,1	
Exercise E	10-12	12,11,11	Z+1	1	1	2,1,2,1	

Remember, only small increments in overload are needed each session and beginners should be able to overload each exercise (especially compounds) frequently.

The first week of a mesocycle does not need to be too intense for a beginner but the last should be, as the next week will be a deload. The proceeding mesocycle after a deload should start at slightly less volume than the end of the previous one, perhaps with as much as the penultimate week before the deload:

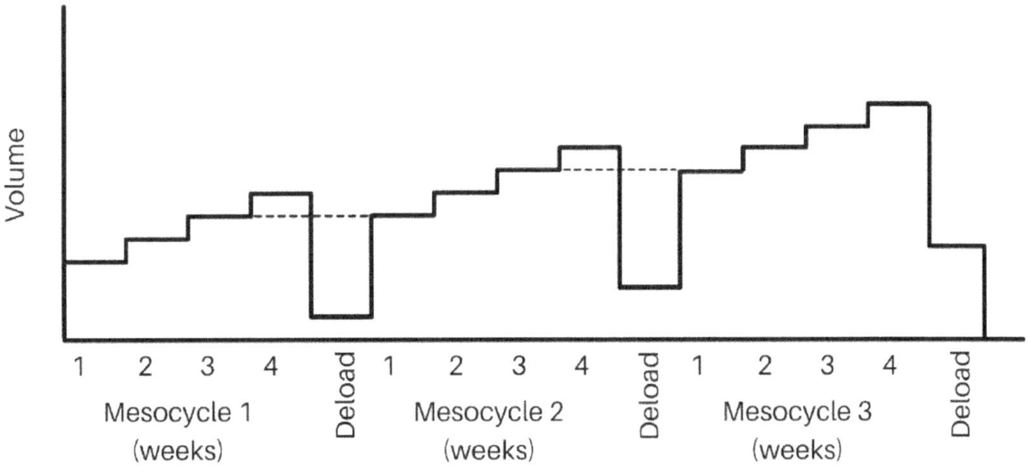

You can see from this graph how the volume progresses over the course of the training programme, creating overload, inducing hypertrophic adaptations.

<u>Exercise execution</u>

Warm ups should not be overlooked. Light aerobic exercise before a workout will warm up muscles, joints and the nervous system, which will optimise training. Note that this shouldn't be cardio training, which will reduce performance of a workout. Warm up sets should be performed prior to working sets for compound exercises and for the first exercise for each muscle group in a workout, to promote good form. It is likely that the isolations won't require warm up sets as compound exercises earlier in the workout will have warmed up the target muscle.

A warm up set should utilise approximately 50% of the working load for at least 5 reps whilst staying well away from failure (at least 4 RIR). Another warmup set of about 75% of the working load could be added, again ensuring to stay well away from failure.

Eg. Warming up for bench press of 3 sets of 8-10 reps of 40kg:

Warm up set 1: Perform about 8 reps of 20kg (50% of working load, which in this case is usually just the bar without plates). Ensure this isn't fatiguing.

Warm up set 2 (optional): Perform about 5 reps of 30kg (75% of working load), again ensuring that this isn't fatiguing.

1) Beginners must be able to perform exercises with good form before adding load. This means taking all movements through a consistent and controlled full range of motion. If a movement is painful, it should be altered or avoided as it will only become more painful as it is overloaded - longevity is key. When learning how to perform exercises, slight differences in technique warranted by individual differences (like angle of foot flare during a squat) are completely acceptable. Some exercises will require more flexibility and mobility than others – choose ones that feel good for you.

2) The most important thing to remember when performing any exercise is that the point of it is to stimulate the target muscle, which means there is no point cheating to lift more weight by recruiting other muscle groups, which will simply cause additional, unnecessary fatigue. Muscle fibres are unaware of how much weight is being lifted, only how much stimulus is being applied to it, so train for muscle stimulus over ego reinforcement – chase stimulus over numbers.

3) Practice does not make perfect; practice makes permanent. Neurological pathways will reinforce the technique performed, so bad form will engrain poor movement patterns.

4) Once exercises can be performed correctly, it is important to keep the performance consistent. It is important not to reduce the range of motion (ROM) or employ bad technique over the course of a set, which is tempting to do as you get closer to failure. Not only will this reduce muscular stimulus, and promote bad movement patterns, but it will also create inconsistencies in tracking. Reps, sets and load are logged to track overload; inconsistencies in rep performance will make it unclear as to whether overload has been progressed, or if some reps have simply been cheated.

5) A good way to review your exercise performance is to film yourself for one or two sets. This will ensure you are not lifting to impress others, with bad technique or going beyond technical failure. Half reps do not count so be honest about when you have hit failure, or if you are closer to it than you think.

6) Conversely however, overthinking technique can distract from exercise execution. All movements should feel natural, so once comfortable with form, the working muscle should be focussed on during execution. There is benefit from deeply focussing on the working muscle in all phases of the movement to fully stimulate it. This neurological pathway, known as "mind muscle connection", should be conscious to beginners.

7) For all exercises, particularly compound and abs exercises, you should inhale during the concentric phase, and exhale during the eccentric phase.

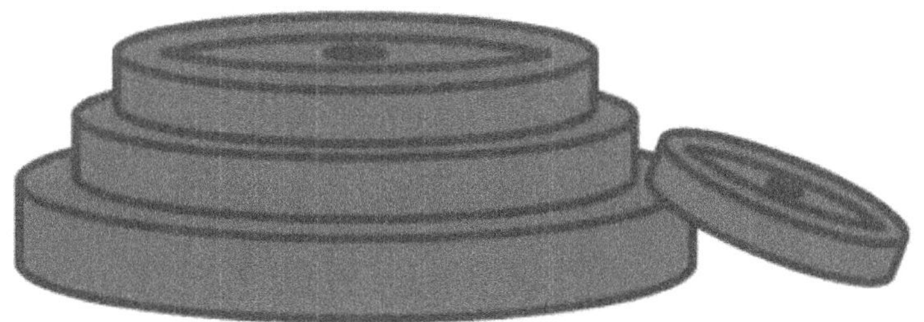

End notes

Training should be fun and enjoyable, and working on your physique should be a rewarding process. The first workout is often the most difficult as it is so stimulating and fatiguing, however as work capacity naturally increases, you will become more comfortable with training, both psychologically and physically.

Finally, for individuals concerned with the daunts of entering a gym for the first time, the best advice is to remember to focus on yourself rather than others around you. The best way to do this is to enter the gym with a plan - a programme. Failing to plan is planning to fail. Every other member in the gym was once a beginner too so focus on you yourself and you'll be making progress in no time.

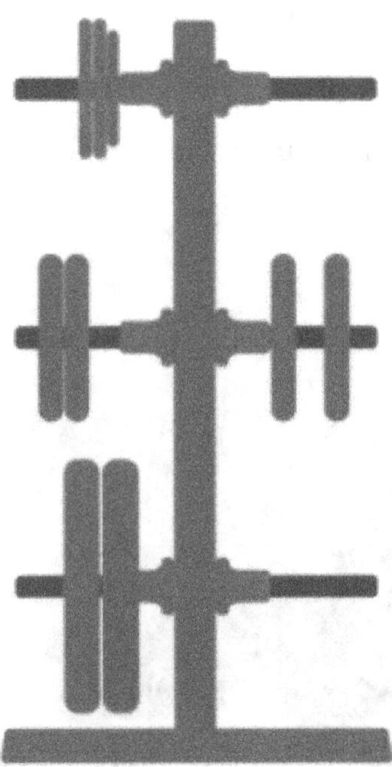

In summary, to make progress in the gym you need a good plan and good execution:

1) Set a specific, personal goal and tailor all aspects of your training to this.

2) Choose exercises that cover the full body to build a balanced physique, focussing on free weight compound movements: vertical and horizontal pulling and pushing, as well as legs.

3) Construct these exercises into a 1-week plan (microcycle) which considers all the training variables. Sustainability should be at the forefront of these considerations.

4) Over the course of the mesocycle, increase volume to create a progressively overloading stimulus to muscles, whilst being mindful of fatigue. Train in the correct rep range, at a high RPE. There is no need to overthink every detail like rest time and tempo – stimulate the target muscles and recover.

5) Record your progress for every set of every exercise and try to improve on this as often as possible.

6) Train with proper form on all exercises; full, consistent ROM (range of motion) without cheating reps by using non-targeted muscle groups.

7) Deload between mesocycles for joint and systemic recovery, which will reduce the risk of injury.

8) Eat and sleep well in conjunction with training

9) Ensure you enjoy your training; take it as seriously as you want but be aware that results are reflective of effort. Alter anything that prevents you from enjoying and sustaining training.

Remember, consistency is key.

Let the gains begin.

Your competition is what you see in the mirror

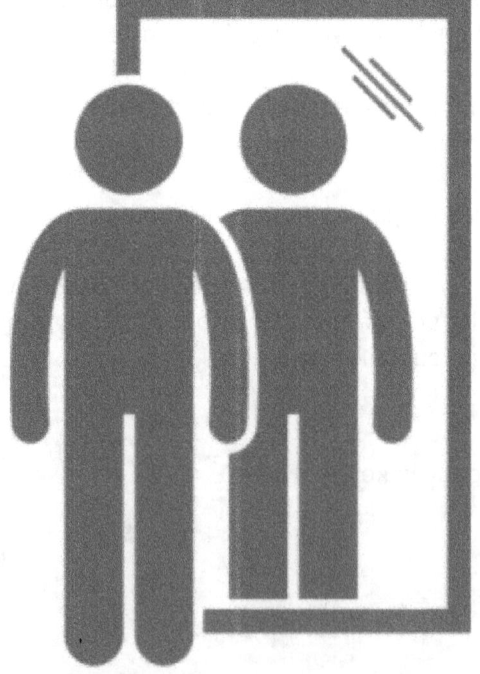

PART 6: Appendices

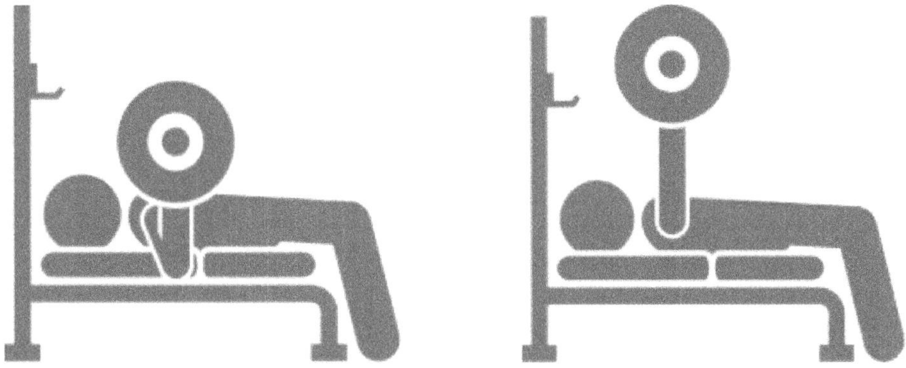

Muscular anatomy

Simple diagrams labelling muscle groups:

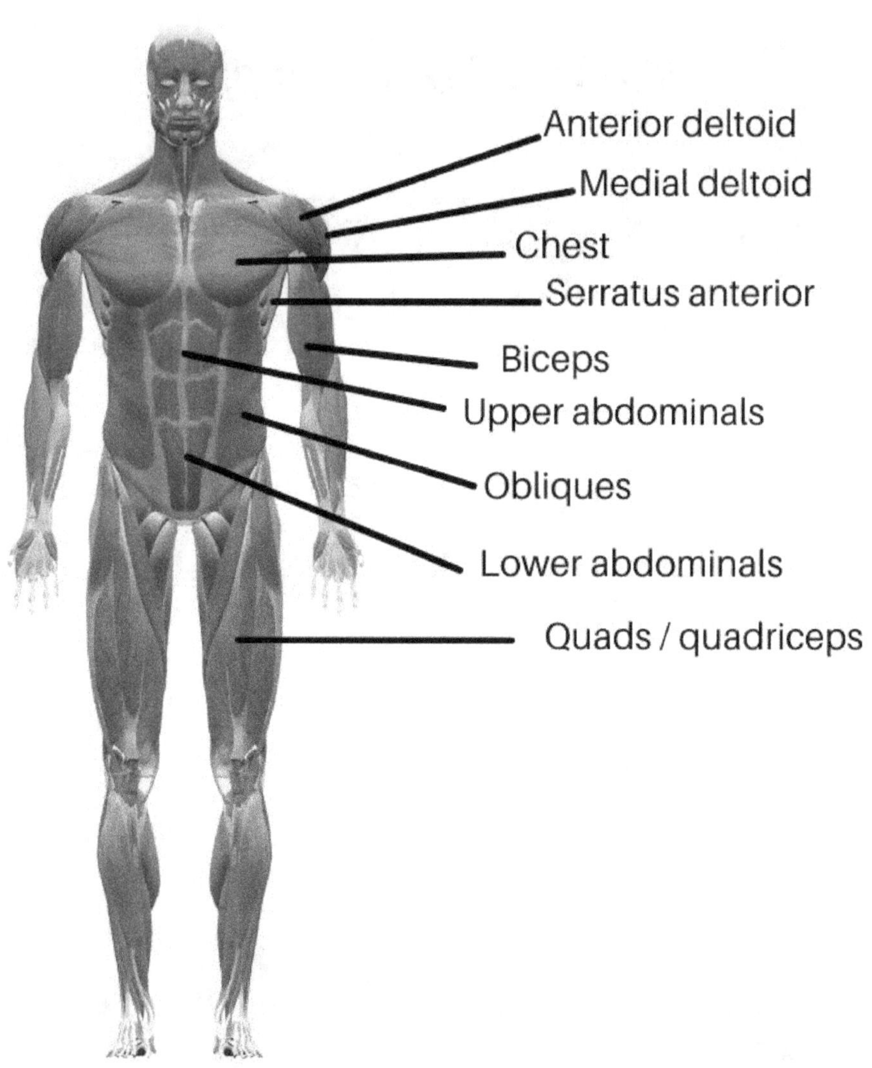

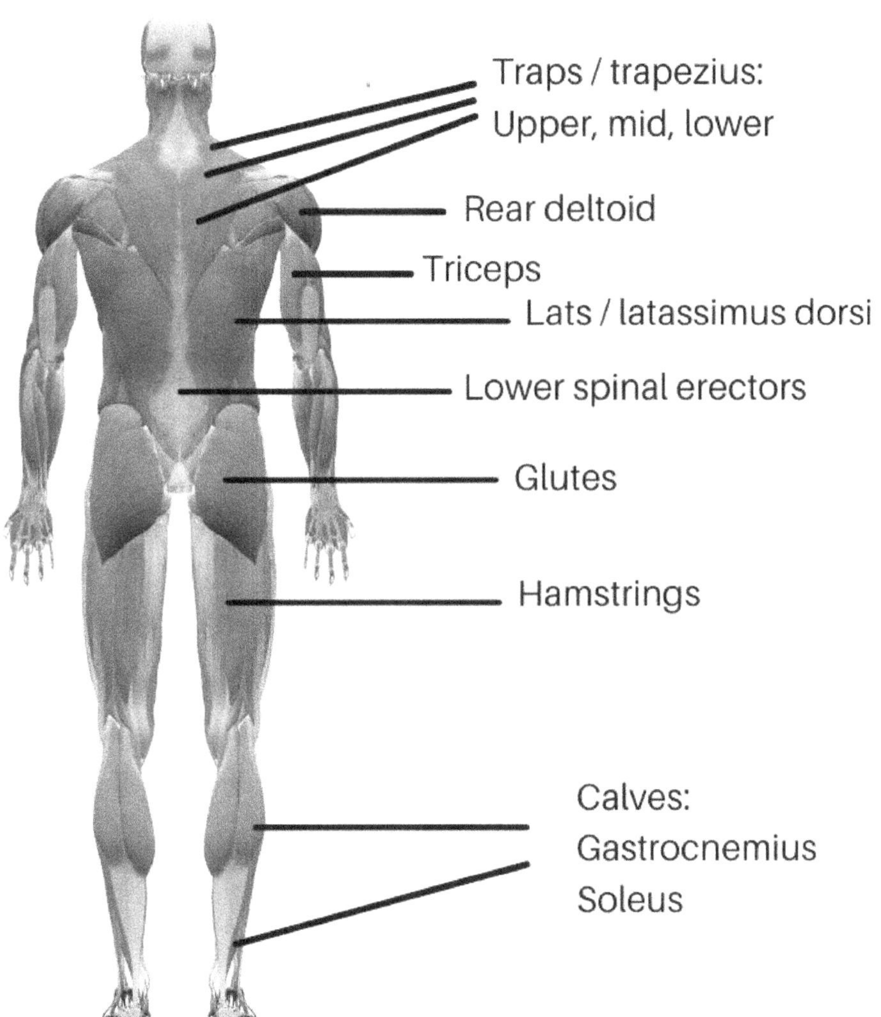

Traps / trapezius:
Upper, mid, lower
Rear deltoid
Triceps
Lats / latassimus dorsi
Lower spinal erectors
Glutes
Hamstrings
Calves:
Gastrocnemius
Soleus

List of exercises

There are hundreds of different exercises and variations, but here is a brief list of some common, recommended exercises, arranged by muscle group.

BB – Barbell

DB – Dumbbell

Chest	BB/DB flat/incline/decline bench press
	Press ups
	Machine chest press
	Dips
	DB/cable flyes

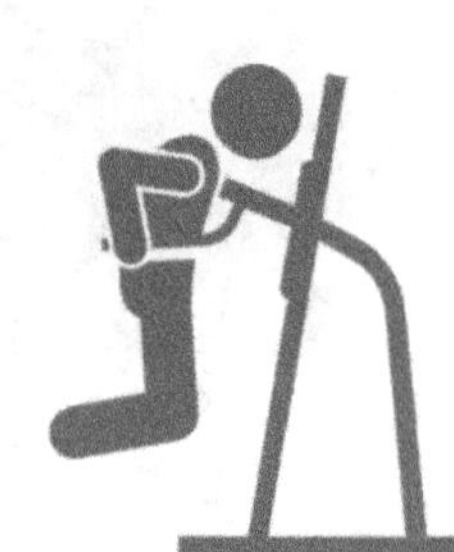

Back (horizontal):	BB/DB bent over row
	BB/DB chest supported row
	T-bar row
	Inverted row
	Cable row

Back (vertical):	Deadlift
	Pull up
	Chin up
	Lat pulldown
	DB pullover
	Cable pullover

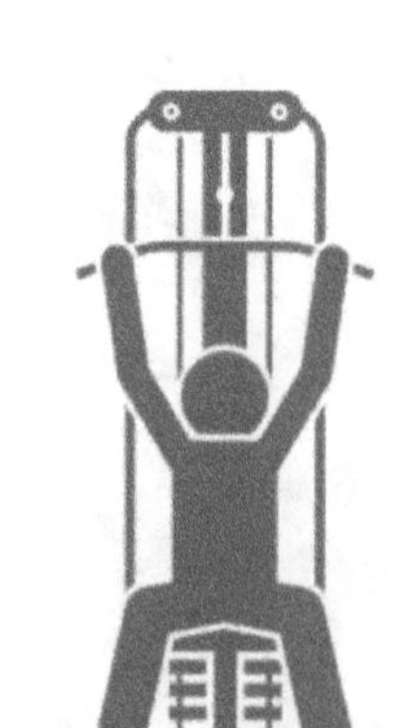

Back (spinal erectors):   Deadlift

Back extensions

Quads: BB back squat (high bar/low bar)

Front squat

Hack squat

Leg press

Lunges

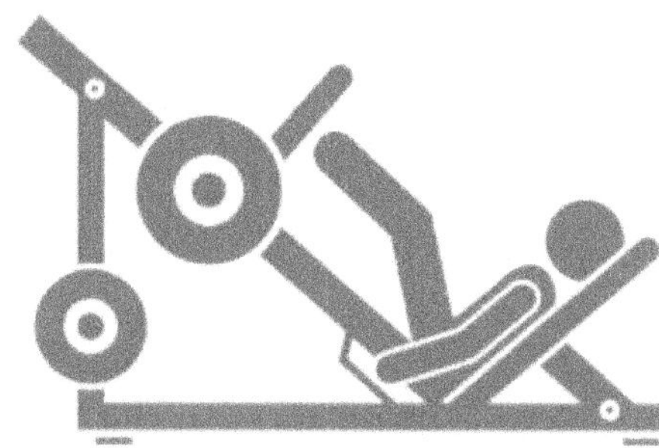

Glutes: Deadlift

BB hip thrust

Lunges

Hamstrings: Stiff-legged deadlift

Good mornings

Prone/seated leg curl

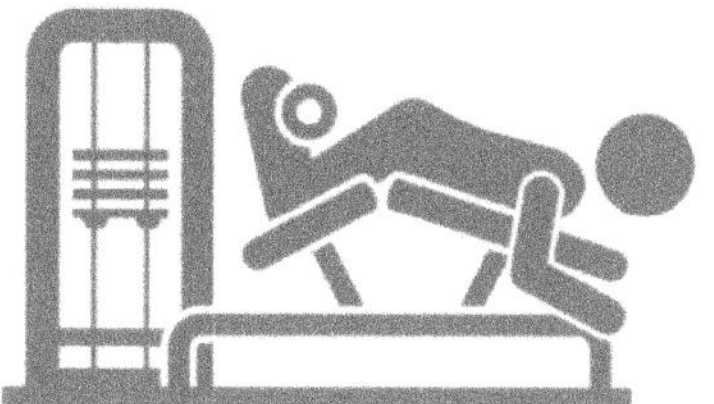

Traps: BB/DB/cable shrug

(often considered part of the back)   Deadlift

Farmer's carry

Also worked during horizontal and vertical pulls

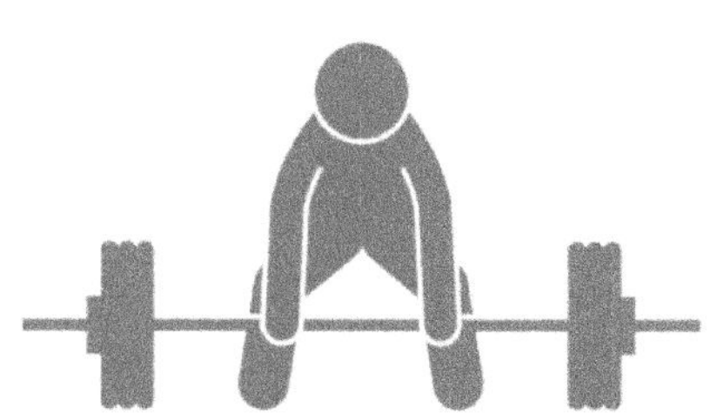

Anterior deltoid: BB/DB OHP

Also worked in horizontal pushes

Medial deltoid: BB/DB OHP

Lateral raises

Rear deltoid: Cable facepull

Bent over DB facepull

Also worked during horizontal and vertical pulling

Triceps: BB/EZ bar skullcrushers

Close group bench press

DB/EZ bar overhead extensions

Cable pushdowns

Overhead rope extensions

Also worked in horizontal and vertical pushes

Biceps: BB/DB/EZ bar/cable curl

Preacher curl

Hammer curl

Also worked in horizontal
and vertical pulls

Forearms: BB wrist curl

DB bench wrist curl

Also worked in horizontal and vertical pulls

Abs:

Supported/hanging leg raises

Cable crunches

Dragonflags

Decline sit ups

Calves:

Seated machine calf raises

Standing calf raise (on leg press machine)

Donkey calf raise

The anterior chain (kinetic chain of anterior muscles groups) opposes the posterior chain (kinetic chain of posterior muscles groups). Muscle groups can be paired with an oppositely functioning muscle group.

Anterior – Posterior:

Chest – Back

Anterior deltoid – posterior deltoid

Biceps – Triceps

Abs – Spinal erectors

Quads – Hamstrings

Hip flexors – Glutes

Other training techniques

Here is a list of training techniques that are beyond the scope of this book. Most of these techniques should only be employed by well-trained intermediate and advanced lifters and should seldom be used by beginners. They are noted here for serious athletes looking to exploit variation in training technique in later years of training:

Supersets

Giant sets

Drop sets

Extreme eccentrics

Sets beyond failure

Pause reps

Blood restriction training

Pyramid and reverse pyramid training

Training with bands and chains

Unilateral training to overcome imbalances in physique

Training different parts of the strength curve for muscular imbalances and overcoming plateaus

Programming more extreme muscle group prioritisation and maintenance

Training muscle groups in different planes of motion to stimulate different fibres; eg. upper chest v lower chest

Training other aspects of fitness like flexibility, mobility, balance, cardio to improve lifting

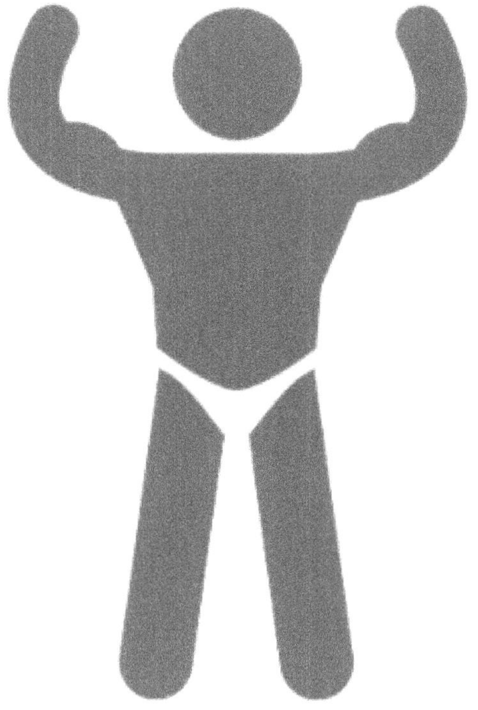